GUIDE ONE:
KNOW YOUR ROOTS
From Root to Tip: A Growing Hands Guide for Natural Hair

BY CONSTANCE HUNTER

For permissions, inquiries, or additional resources, please contact:

Pre'Vail Natural Hair Salon

www.prevailyournatural.com | prevailyournatural@gmail.com

This book is intended for informational and educational purposes only and should serve as a general guide to understanding and improving natural hair health. While the methods and recommendations provided are based on expertise in natural hair care and trichology, they are not intended to replace professional medical or dermatological advice.

If you are experiencing severe scalp conditions, excessive hair loss, or other persistent issues, it is strongly recommended that you consult a licensed dermatologist or a professional cosmetologist specializing in scalp and hair health. A trained professional can assess underlying causes and provide personalized treatment plans tailored to your specific needs.

By using the information in this book, the reader acknowledges that the author and publisher are not responsible for individual outcomes. Readers should exercise their own discretion when applying the suggested practices.

First Edition: 2025

ISBN

PaperBack: 978-1-968134-01-3

Ebook: 978-1-968134-10-5

Printed in USA

ABOUT THE AUTHOR

As a certified trichologist and natural hair care educator, I specialize in helping individuals discover what's truly possible for their hair—especially when they've been told otherwise.

My passion lies in witnessing transformation—that moment when someone realizes their hair can be healthy, strong, and free. With a deep understanding of the science behind hair and scalp health, I strive to provide clarity, comfort, and actionable solutions. My training equips me to assess and guide care for a wide range of concerns, from common challenges like dandruff and dryness to complex conditions such as alopecia areata, scalp psoriasis, and CCCA.

But my work goes beyond diagnosis or technique. I believe in education, empowerment, and helping clients build routines that nourish their crown from root to tip. This includes learning to read labels, choosing products with purpose, avoiding harmful styling practices, and embracing care that fits their lifestyle and values.

While I offer expert insight from the field of trichology, I'm not a medical doctor. Hair and scalp symptoms can sometimes signal deeper health issues. That's why I encourage a holistic approach—and, when necessary, consulting licensed healthcare professionals for comprehensive support.

In this series, you'll find guidance rooted in science, experience, and care. My hope is that it not only helps you understand your hair better but also love it more, trust it more, and grow with it in ways you never thought possible.

Your hair is not the problem—you just needed the right guide.

DEDICATION

For the one just starting to ask,
"What if my hair was never the problem?"

This is your beginning.

You are not broken.

You just need to know.

OVERVIEW

Your natural hair journey begins with understanding. *Know Your Roots* sets the foundation by helping you reconnect with the true structure, science, and beauty of your natural hair. This guide clears the confusion around curl patterns, porosity, and texture—and replaces it with clarity, care, and confidence.

Whether you're just starting your natural journey or years in and still figuring it out, this guide gives you the knowledge you never got—but always needed.

SERIES INTRODUCTION

Welcome to *From Root to Tip: A Growing Hands Guide for Natural Hair*

This series was created with one goal in mind: to give you what's been missing—not just products, not just trends, but truth, support, and real guidance for real people who are ready to finally understand and care for their natural hair from the inside out.

For years, we've been taught to manage, fix, or fight our hair. But here, we're doing something different. We're returning to care—not control. To confidence. To consistency. To choice.

Each guide in this series is built as a step in your journey. They can be read in order or on their own, depending on where you are in your process. Whether you're just starting out, rebuilding your relationship with your hair, or deepening your understanding, this space is for you.

I've written these guides from my hands—growing hands that have touched, healed, protected, and restored countless crowns. Now, I offer that care to you.

This isn't just about hair. It's about healing. It's about reclaiming your rhythm, your confidence, and your beauty—from root to tip.

Let's begin.

WHAT YOU WILL LEARN

- What "natural hair" really means—beyond the buzzwords

- The structure of a strand: follicle, shaft, and cuticle

- How to identify your curl pattern, density, and porosity

- Why porosity matters more than curl type

- The impact of myths, media, and misinformation on how we treat our hair

- A beginner's approach to honoring your texture with care, not control

WHAT YOU'LL WALK AWAY WITH

- A clear understanding of your hair type and its unique needs

- The confidence to stop chasing trends and start trusting your texture

- The mindset to treat your hair as something sacred—not something to fix

- A solid foundation for building your care, style, and healing routine

TABLE OF CONTENTS

INTRODUCTION

This isn't about hair types and trends. It's about truth.

For too long, you've been told your hair is *difficult*, *unprofessional*, or something to fix. But the truth is, your hair isn't the problem—*misunderstanding is.*

In **Guide One**, we go back to the beginning—not just to your roots physically, but emotionally and culturally. We explore how natural hair has been misunderstood for generations and give you the language and insight to break that cycle. You'll learn to see your hair clearly—its density, porosity, and curl pattern—and finally understand how to care for it *your way.*

This guide is your introduction to a new relationship with your hair—rooted in knowledge and growing in love.

LESSON 1:
EMBRACING THE BEAUTY AND DIVERSITY OF NATURAL TEXTURED HAIR

Afro-textured hair, often referred to as natural hair, embodies a rich history, deep cultural significance, and undeniable beauty. This lesson introduces the incredible uniqueness of natural textured hair and highlights the importance of celebrating its beauty and diversity. For far too long, natural hair faced unfair scrutiny, was misunderstood, and was marginalized by mainstream society. However, today, the natural hair movement has ignited a wave of pride and celebration for Afro-textured hair, honoring its originality, versatility, and representation of cultural identity.

Natural textured hair is as diverse as the people who wear it—no two heads of hair are exactly alike. While there are specific classifications for curl types, natural hair varies in density, porosity, and curl patterns, which can differ even on the same head. This diversity allows for a stunning array of hairstyles and expressions of individuality. For many, learning to love and embrace their natural hair is an essential part of personal growth and self-acceptance.

Through this lesson, we'll explore the beauty of natural hair, delve into its historical and cultural roots, and understand why embracing it is an empowering act of self-love, rebellion, and affirmation.

Celebrating the Uniqueness of Natural Textured Hair

One of the most beautiful aspects of Afro-textured hair is its individuality. Whether your curls are tightly coiled, loose, or somewhere in between, natural hair is uniquely yours. It allows for a level of creativity and versatility that many other hair types simply do not offer. From afros to braids, twists, and protective styles, the possibilities for self-expression are endless.

The natural hair movement, which began gaining prominence in the early 2000s, has played a vital role in reclaiming the narrative surrounding Afro-textured hair. It became a platform for embracing the beauty of natural hair in its authentic state, encouraging individuals to reject harmful beauty standards that promoted straightening or altering hair to conform to Eurocentric ideals. By choosing to wear natural hair in all its textured glory, individuals send a powerful message: beauty comes in all forms.

The variety within natural hair types is part of what makes it so special. Afro-textured hair is often classified by curl patterns, grouped into categories ranging from 3A to 4C. While 3A hair typically features looser curls, 4C hair—one of the tightest curl patterns—forms small, dense coils. Though this scale is widely recognized, it has its limitations. Many textures fall between categories, and the numbers can be confusing. Charting by shrinkage percentage offers an alternative that may more accurately identify textures. Each type of curl brings its own unique set of challenges and beauty, and learning how to care for your specific hair type is an essential part of embracing it fully.

Flowing Curls   Gentle Curls   Springy Coils   Tight Corkscrews   Zigzag Kinks

Hair Shrinkage Scale

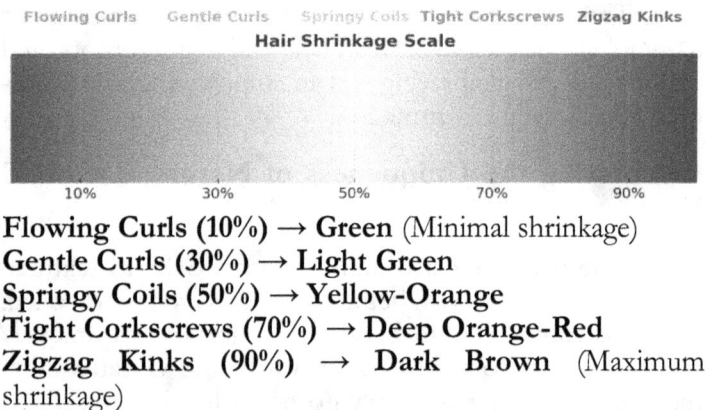

10%   30%   50%   70%   90%

Flowing Curls (10%) → **Green** (Minimal shrinkage)
Gentle Curls (30%) → **Light Green**
Springy Coils (50%) → **Yellow-Orange**
Tight Corkscrews (70%) → **Deep Orange-Red**
Zigzag Kinks (90%) → **Dark Brown** (Maximum shrinkage)

Shrinkage-Based Hair Texture Scale

Shrinkage	Image	Name	Strand Thickness	Description	Porosity
10-20%		Gentle Curls (2A-2C)	Fine/ Medium	Hair retains most of its stretched length with slight curling or bending, forming soft, loose wave patterns.	Moisture-Resistant (Hair repels water and takes time to absorb products)
30-40%		Flowing Curls (3A-3B)	Fine / Medium / Coarse	Hair shrinks moderately, with curls forming more defined spirals but still maintaining noticeable length.	Moisture-Resistant to Balanced Absorption (Gradually absorbs moisture but retains it well)
50-60%		Springy Coils (3C-4A)	Medium / Coarse	Hair has a balanced mix of shrinkage and elongation, with well-defined curls or coils.	Balanced Absorption to Moisture-Absorbent (Holds moisture well but may need extra hydration)
70-80%		Tight Corkscrews (4A-4B)	Medium / Coarse	Hair shrinks significantly, forming tighter, springy coils that lose a large portion of their stretched length.	Moisture-Absorbent but Fast-Drying (Absorbs water quickly but needs sealing products to retain moisture)
90-100%		Zigzag Kinks (4B-4C)	Coarse	Hair experiences maximum shrinkage, forming densely packed kinks or zigzag patterns that retain little of their stretched length.	Highly Moisture-Absorbent but Fast- Drying (Loses moisture rapidly and requires frequent hydration)

Beyond its physical appearance, natural hair is often a reflection of personality, self-expression, and confidence. For many people with Afro-textured hair, it is far more than just a physical feature—it is a symbol of pride, culture, and identity. The decision to embrace natural hair often follows a journey of self-discovery, where individuals learn to appreciate the inherent beauty of their hair, free from societal expectations or judgments.

Historical Context of Natural Hair

To truly appreciate the beauty and significance of natural textured hair, we must explore its historical context. Afro-textured hair has been deeply intertwined with cultural identity for centuries, long before colonization and the imposition of European beauty standards.

In ancient African civilizations, hair was much more than a physical feature—it was a symbol of status, spirituality, and identity. Different hairstyles were used to signify one's tribe, social standing, marital status, age, wealth, and even fertility. Braiding patterns, in particular, were often passed down through generations, serving as a means to communicate heritage. In some cultures, intricate braiding patterns were reserved for religious rituals or special ceremonies, highlighting the sacred role of hair in African societies.

However, the transatlantic slave trade and colonization drastically altered the perception and significance of natural hair. Enslaved Africans were stripped of their cultural practices, including the hairstyling traditions that had been central to their communities. Hair, once a source of pride and identity, became a target of shame as European colonizers imposed beauty standards centered around straight hair textures. Deprived of the tools and products needed to care for their hair, many enslaved individuals resorted to covering it with scarves or rags to conceal its natural state.

As Africans were forcibly brought to the Americas, the suppression of natural hair's beauty and cultural importance intensified. European colonizers equated straight hair with cleanliness, professionalism, and respectability, while Afro-textured hair was stigmatized as inferior and unkempt. This bias gave rise to the widespread use of chemical relaxers, hot combs, and other methods aimed at straightening or altering natural hair to conform to these rigid and exclusionary beauty standards.

The Role of Hair in the Civil Rights Movement

Despite immense pressure to conform to European beauty standards, Afro-textured hair has long served as a powerful tool of resistance and self-expression. During the Civil Rights Movement of the 1960s and 1970s, natural hair became a symbol of Black pride and political activism. The iconic Afro hairstyle, worn by activists like Angela Davis, came to embody the fight for equality and justice. Choosing to wear natural hair in its unaltered state was an act of defiance against a system that had historically devalued Black bodies and Black beauty.

The Afro, in particular, symbolized a rejection of assimilation and an embrace of Black identity. For many, wearing their hair naturally was a radical statement, an assertion that Black was beautiful. The natural hair movement of the 1960s encouraged African Americans to reconnect with their cultural roots and resist societal pressures dictating how they should present themselves.

However, even during this time of empowerment, Afro-textured hair was not fully embraced by mainstream society. Many workplaces and schools enforced strict grooming policies that prohibited natural hairstyles, perpetuating the idea that natural hair was unprofessional. The fight to normalize and accept natural hair was far from over.

Cultural Significance of Natural Hair Today

Fast forward to the present day, and the significance of natural hair continues to evolve. The natural hair movement of the 21st century, largely fueled by social media, has ushered in a new wave of empowerment for those with Afro-textured hair. Platforms like YouTube, Instagram, and Twitter have become hubs where natural hair enthusiasts share tips, tutorials, and product recommendations, fostering a supportive community for individuals navigating their natural hair journeys.

Today, embracing natural hair goes beyond rejecting Eurocentric beauty standards—it's about reclaiming autonomy over one's appearance and challenging the notion that straight hair is the only "professional" or "acceptable" hair type. Celebrities, influencers, and everyday individuals proudly showcase their natural hair, helping to normalize the rich diversity of hairstyles and textures that fall under the umbrella of Afro-textured hair.

For many, the decision to transition from chemically relaxed or heat-damaged hair to natural hair is deeply personal. It often represents a journey of self-love, self-acceptance, and a reconnection with cultural heritage. Embracing natural hair is about far more than aesthetics; it is an act of rejecting years of internalized shame and celebrating the beauty of individuality.

The natural hair movement has also driven meaningful legislative change. In the United States, for instance, the Crown Act (Creating a Respectful and Open World for Natural Hair) has been enacted in several states to prohibit discrimination based on hair texture or protective styles like braids and locs. This legislation underscores the ongoing fight for acceptance and equal treatment of natural hair in schools, workplaces, and public spaces.

Embracing Your Natural Hair

Learning to embrace natural hair is a journey that requires education, patience, and self- compassion. For many, growing up with natural hair meant hearing that it was too difficult to manage, too "wild," or too unprofessional. As a result, many turned to relaxers, weaves, and wigs in an attempt to conform to societal standards.

However, transitioning to natural hair can be a liberating experience. It's an opportunity to unlearn years of negative conditioning and embrace the beauty of your natural texture. It's about rejecting the idea that your hair needs to be "fixed" and understanding that it is perfect just as it is.

Embracing natural hair is also a way to take ownership of your self-expression. Your hair becomes a canvas for creativity, whether you choose to wear it in an afro, braids, twists, or a protective style. Each hairstyle tells a unique story and represents a part of your identity.

At its core, embracing natural textured hair is an act of love—love for yourself, your heritage, and your individuality.

LESSON 2:
HAIR STRUCTURE AND TYPES

Understanding Natural Textured Hair Structure and Types

To effectively care for natural textured hair, it's essential to understand its structure and the various types. Natural hair, particularly Afro-textured hair, is unique in its complexity, resilience, and beauty. However, these distinct qualities can sometimes make it seem challenging to manage without the right knowledge. By understanding the structure of hair and recognizing its different types, you can identify the best care methods for maintaining healthy hair. This lesson will explore the anatomy of the hair strand and explain the classification system for different hair types, with a focus on types 4A, 4B, and 4C.

1. The Cuticle

The outermost layer of the hair strand is called the cuticle. It consists of overlapping, scale-like cells that protect the inner structure of the hair. In healthy hair, the cuticle lies flat, creating a smooth surface that reflects light and gives the hair a shiny appearance. In textured hair, the cuticle layers tend to lift more easily due to the natural bends and curves in the hair. This can make textured hair more prone to dryness and damage if not properly cared for. The raised cuticle also means that natural hair requires more moisture, not protein, to maintain elasticity and reduce breakage.

2. The Cortex

The cortex is the middle layer of the hair strand, where the strength, elasticity, and color of the hair are determined. It consists of fibrous proteins (primarily keratin) that provide the hair with its structure. The arrangement of these proteins varies across different hair types and largely determines the hair's texture, thickness, and curl pattern. In natural textured hair, the proteins in the cortex are coiled more tightly, contributing to the hair's distinctive curl patterns. This makes the hair more fragile due to its inherent twists and turns.

3. The Medulla

The innermost part of the hair strand is the medulla. It's a soft, spongy core that may be absent in some hair types, particularly fine or thin hair. The medulla's exact function is not fully understood, but it is believed to provide some insulation to the hair strand. In thicker and coarser hair types, including many forms of Afro-textured hair, the medulla is more likely to be present.

The Importance of Hair Porosity

In addition to the basic structure of the hair strand, it's important to understand hair porosity, which refers to how well your hair can absorb and retain moisture. Porosity plays a significant role in how natural hair reacts to products, moisture, and styling. Hair porosity is typically categorized into three levels:

Low porosity: Hair with low porosity has tightly packed cuticle layers, making it difficult for moisture to penetrate. This type of hair may feel heavy and resist products like oils or creams. However, once moisture is absorbed, it tends to retain it well.

Medium (normal) porosity: Hair with medium porosity absorbs and retains moisture effectively. It typically responds well to styling products and holds moisture without becoming overly dry or greasy.

High porosity: Hair with high porosity has raised cuticles, allowing moisture to enter easily but making it difficult to retain. High porosity hair is more prone to frizz and dryness, and while it absorbs products quickly, it may lose moisture just as fast.

Natural textured hair tends to be more porous, especially if it has been chemically treated or heat-styled frequently. This can lead to dryness and an increased need for added moisture.

Differentiating between Hair Types (e.g., 4A, 4B, 4C)

The texture and type of natural hair are often classified using a system of numbers and letters to describe curl patterns. To assist with this, we'll also use the shrinkage percentage scale I created, which will help you correctly identify your hair type. This classification system is crucial for understanding the specific needs of each hair type, allowing you to choose the right products and care techniques. While there are several types of curls, types 4A, 4B, and 4C are most commonly associated with natural Afro-textured hair. These hair types are characterized by their tightly coiled curl patterns and require particular attention to hydration, detangling, and protective styling.

1. Type 4A Hair 60-70%

Type 4A hair features a tight, defined curl pattern that resembles an "S" shape when stretched. These curls are usually well-defined and can be easily seen without manipulation. Type 4A hair tends to be softer in texture and retains more moisture than the other type 4 categories, but it can still become dry and fragile without proper care.

Because the curls are tightly coiled, it's essential to maintain moisture with hydrating products such as leave-in conditioners, creams, and natural oils. The curl pattern in 4A hair also allows for versatile styling options, including wash-and-go styles and twist-outs, which help retain curl definition and minimize frizz.

2. Type 4B Hair 70-80%

Type 4B hair features a more tightly coiled pattern than 4A, with curls forming a distinct "Z" shape. The sharp angles in 4B hair result in a less defined curl pattern, making it more prone to shrinkage and dryness. The strands often have a cotton-like texture, and the dense coils can cause the hair to appear shorter than its actual length.

4B hair is highly versatile and lends itself to a wide range of styling options, but it requires a careful balance of moisture to remain healthy. Regular deep conditioning treatments, combined with protective styles like braids or twists, are essential for preventing breakage and retaining moisture. Preventing tangles is a key part of 4B hair care, as the zigzag pattern of the curls makes it prone to knotting. To maintain healthy hair, regular trims—recommended at least every quarter—are crucial.

3. Type 4C Hair 80% and higher

Type 4C hair is the most tightly coiled of all curl types. Its curl pattern is less defined compared to 4A and 4B, and it often experiences significant shrinkage—over 80% of its actual length. This hair type requires the most moisture and care, as it is particularly prone to breakage due to its fragility and density.

The tightly coiled strands are more susceptible to tangling and dryness, making frequent moisturizing with water-based products—such as leave-ins, moisturizers, and creams— essential. Regular deep conditioning and protective styles are vital for maintaining the health of 4C hair, as they help lock in moisture and minimize damage.

The high level of shrinkage makes styles like twist-outs, braid-outs, or stretched styles popular among those with 4C hair. These styles not only elongate the curls but also showcase the hair's true length.

Curl Pattern and Hair Care

Understanding your hair's curl pattern is the first step toward building a healthy hair care routine. Natural hair types, particularly those in the 4A to 4C range, require moisture-rich products tailored to their unique needs. Here are some general tips for caring for natural textured hair based on its structure and type:

1. Moisture is Key

All types of natural hair benefit from moisture, but tightly coiled hair tends to lose hydration more quickly than looser curl patterns. Regular use of water-based moisturizers and leave-in conditioners helps retain moisture. It's equally important to seal in that moisture with heavier oils or butters, such as shea butter or castor oil.

Keep in mind: Oil does not provide moisture. It seals in moisture and, if not used correctly, can even block moisture from penetrating the hair.

2. Gentle Detangling

Tight curl patterns, like those in types 4A to 4C, require careful detangling to minimize breakage. A detangling paddle brush (such as "The Unbrush") is one of the simplest and most effective tools for protecting your hair during this process. Pair it with a good detangling product to make the task easier and to reduce damage.

While finger detangling can assist during the process, it does not effectively remove all shed hair. Over time, this can weaken the hair and lead to more breakage. Using your fingers as a supplementary tool is fine, but always finish with a brush to ensure thorough detangling.

3. Protective Styling

Protective styles, such as braids, twists, and updos, are essential for reducing manipulation and preventing breakage, especially for type 4B and 4C hair. These styles protect the ends of your hair, the oldest and most fragile part, while also promoting growth and moisture retention. Be sure to prep your hair before styling by trimming and deep conditioning, allowing your hair to rest in its best condition for the style.

4. Regular Deep Conditioning

Deep conditioning treatments are vital for maintaining the health of natural hair, especially for types 4A, 4B, and 4C. Using a moisturizing deep conditioner once a week helps restore hydration and strengthens the hair shaft. It's important to avoid excessive protein treatments, as most hair struggles with moisture depletion rather than a lack of strength. Moisture is the key to preventing and reducing breakage.

5. Avoid Excessive Heat

Excessive heat can damage natural hair by breaking down the proteins that provide its structure. Limit the use of heat styling tools, such as flat irons and blow dryers. When heat is necessary, always apply a heat protectant. Use low to medium heat, and ensure your flat iron and blow dryer are smokeless to prevent hair damage.

Understanding the structure of natural textured hair and recognizing the differences between various curl patterns is crucial for maintaining healthy hair. Each hair type within the type 4 category—4A, 4B, and 4C—has unique characteristics and care needs. By learning about your specific hair type and curl pattern, you can create a hair care routine that promotes moisture retention, reduces breakage, and enhances the natural beauty of your hair.

Embrace the versatility and uniqueness of your natural hair, and remember: healthy hair is beautiful hair!

LESSON 3:
COMMON HAIR MYTHS AND MISCONCEPTIONS

For centuries, Afro-textured hair has been surrounded by myths, stereotypes, and misconceptions. These misunderstandings have influenced societal perceptions of natural hair and shaped how individuals with Afro hair view and care for their tresses. Rooted in historical biases or a lack of understanding, these myths have contributed to the marginalization and misrepresentation of the beauty and diversity of Afro-textured hair.

This lesson aims to debunk some of the most common myths about Afro hair by providing science-based insights and challenging long-held stereotypes. Embracing the truth about Afro hair is a crucial step toward healthier, more empowered hair care practices and celebrating the beauty and versatility of natural hair.

Challenging Stereotypes and Misconceptions

1. Myth: Afro Hair Doesn't Grow Long

One of the most pervasive myths about Afro-textured hair is the belief that it doesn't grow as long as other hair types. This misconception likely arises from the coiled structure of Afro hair, which causes shrinkage, making the hair appear shorter than its actual length.

In reality, all hair types grow at approximately the same rate—about half an inch to an inch per month on average. The key difference lies in length retention. Due to its tightly coiled structure, Afro hair is more fragile and prone to breakage, which can make retaining length more challenging.

Shrinkage, a natural characteristic of curly and coily hair, is often mistaken for a lack of growth. However, shrinkage is a sign of healthy hair elasticity and should be celebrated. Proper care, knowledge, and patience can help Afro hair thrive and grow long. The key to achieving length lies in reducing breakage and focusing on retaining the length of existing strands through gentle care and protective practices.

2. Myth: Afro Hair Is Naturally Tough and Strong

Another common misconception is that Afro hair is inherently strong and durable due to its dense and thick appearance. While it may seem robust, Afro-textured hair is actually one of the most fragile hair types.

The tight curls and coils create multiple points of tension along the hair shaft, making Afro hair more prone to breakage, especially when exposed to friction, harsh styling, or heat.

Additionally, Afro hair has a raised cuticle structure, allowing moisture to escape more easily. This leaves the hair dry and susceptible to damage.

Afro hair requires gentle care and should not be treated as though it can withstand more force or manipulation than other hair types. Incorporating protective styles, practicing low manipulation techniques, and maintaining consistent moisture are essential steps for preserving the health and strength of Afro hair.

3. Myth: Washing Afro Hair Frequently Is Bad for It

One of the most prevalent myths about Afro hair is that frequent washing leads to dryness or breakage. While it's true that Afro-textured hair tends to be drier than other hair types, this doesn't mean it should be washed infrequently. Skipping regular washes can cause product buildup, scalp irritation, and even stunted hair growth. The primary goal of shampooing is to cleanse the scalp, ensuring it gets the oxygen it needs to stay healthy.

The key isn't to avoid washing but to use moisturizing shampoos and conditioners that hydrate the hair without stripping its natural oils. Cleansing and detox shampoos are rarely recommended for Afro hair. Additionally, using lukewarm water instead of hot water during washes helps prevent excessive dryness.

As a general guideline, washing Afro hair every two weeks works well for many individuals. However, this frequency can be adjusted based on personal preference, hair condition, and styling routines.

4. Myth: Natural Hair Doesn't Need Trimming

Another common misconception is that trimming natural Afro hair prevents it from growing long or that trims aren't necessary. In reality, regular trims are essential for maintaining healthy hair, regardless of texture. Afro hair is particularly prone to split ends and breakage, which, if left untrimmed, can travel up the hair shaft and cause further damage.

Trimming every 8 to 12 weeks helps remove damaged ends, reduce tangling, and improve overall hair health. While trims won't make hair grow faster, they do prevent breakage, allowing hair to retain length over time. Regular trims should be seen as a vital part of a healthy hair care routine, not as an obstacle to growth.

In fact, you're likely to lose more hair to breakage than you would from a trim. When done regularly and paired with proper moisture maintenance, trims typically require removing just an inch or less of hair at a time.

5. Myth: Afro Hair Can't Be Versatile

Afro-textured hair is often stereotyped as difficult to style or lacking versatility, but nothing could be further from the truth. Natural hair is one of the most versatile types, offering a wide range of styling options—from afros and twist-outs to braids, locs, and protective updos. It can be worn straight, curly, or styled into countless creative looks, depending on how it's treated and manipulated.

Protective styles such as braids, twists, and cornrows are especially popular, as they safeguard the hair while allowing for diverse and creative aesthetics. The versatility of Afro hair highlights its uniqueness and provides endless opportunities for self-expression.

The misconception that Afro hair is difficult to manage or style often stems from a lack of understanding about proper care practices and the right products to use.

6. Myth: Afro Hair Requires Relaxers to Be Manageable

For many years, chemical relaxers were marketed as the only solution for managing Afro- textured hair, perpetuating the myth that natural hair is unmanageable in its untreated state. This misconception was reinforced by societal pressures to conform to Eurocentric beauty standards, which often favored straight hair over textured hair.

In reality, natural Afro hair is entirely manageable with the right care routine, products, and techniques. Relaxers, which chemically straighten the hair, can cause significant long-term damage, including thinning, breakage, and scalp irritation. Moreover, many women of color experience Central Centrifugal Cicatricial Alopecia (CCCA), a condition that can be triggered or worsened by the use of relaxers.

Today, a growing number of individuals have embraced their natural hair texture, finding that with proper moisturizing, detangling, and protective styling, their hair can be both manageable and healthy. Caring for Afro hair does not require harsh chemicals—just an understanding of how to nourish and protect its unique texture.

7.   Myth: Afro Hair Needs to Be Greased Daily

The tradition of applying hair grease or heavy oils to Afro hair daily has been passed down through generations but is rooted in a misunderstanding of how to properly moisturize natural hair. While Afro hair does require more moisture than straighter hair types, grease and heavy oils are not effective for hydration. Instead, they can create a barrier that blocks moisture from penetrating the hair shaft, leading to dryness and product buildup when overused.

Rather than greasing the hair, these products are better suited for occasional use on the scalp— no more than once or twice a week and always in moderation. This helps avoid clogging the scalp or weighing down the hair. For maintaining hydration, sealing in moisture with natural oils like jojoba or argan oil is a much more effective approach.

Science-Based Insights on Natural Hair Care

Now that we've debunked common myths about Afro hair, let's explore the science behind natural hair care. Understanding the biology of Afro-textured hair empowers us to create healthier routines based on facts rather than misconceptions.

1.   The Importance of Moisture for Afro Hair

The coiled structure of Afro hair makes it challenging for natural scalp oils (sebum) to travel down the hair shaft, leaving the hair naturally drier than other types. Science confirms that keeping Afro hair moisturized is essential for maintaining elasticity, reducing breakage, and promoting overall health.

Water-based moisturizers, deep conditioning treatments, and hydrating leave-in conditioners are key for keeping Afro hair soft, supple, and resilient.

2. Protein Treatments for Strength

Hair is primarily composed of keratin, a protein, which makes protein treatments an important part of maintaining hair health. However, Afro-textured hair generally benefits more from moisture than protein since dryness is often the primary cause of breakage.

Excessive protein use, especially on chemically treated or heat-styled hair, can lead to brittleness and worsen dryness. For the best results, protein treatments should always be balanced with moisturizing treatments to achieve a healthy moisture-protein balance.

3. Gentle Detangling to Prevent Breakage

Because of its coiled structure, Afro hair is prone to tangles and knots, making gentle detangling crucial to prevent unnecessary breakage. Detangling works best on damp or conditioned hair, as this minimizes stress on the strands.

However, wet hair is more fragile, so it's essential to detangle carefully, using the right tools and techniques. This protects the hair's integrity and minimizes damage, ensuring healthier, stronger hair over time.

QUIZ

Lesson 1: Embracing the Beauty and Diversity of Natural Textured Hair

1. Question

What are some reasons why natural textured hair is celebrated in today's society?

a) It is versatile and allows for a variety of styles.

b) It has strong cultural and historical significance.

c) It is easier to manage than straight hair.

d) Both a and b.

Answer: d) Both a and b.

2. Question

During which historical period did natural hair become a symbol of Black pride and resistance?

a) The Civil Rights Movement.

b) The Industrial Revolution.

c) World War II.

d) The Renaissance.

Answer: a) The Civil Rights Movement.

3. Question

Which of the following is NOT a benefit of embracing natural hair?

a) Celebrating your natural beauty.

b) Reducing heat damage.

c) Needing fewer hair products.

d) Improving self-confidence.

Answer: c) Needing fewer hair products.

Lesson 2: Hair Structure and Types

1. Question

What is the key characteristic that differentiates hair types like 4A, 4B, and 4C?

a) The hair's thickness.

b) The curl pattern.

c) The length of the hair.

d) The color of the hair.

Answer: b) The curl pattern.

2. Question

Which of the following best describes hair porosity?

a) The way hair absorbs and retains moisture.

b) The length of hair.

c) The thickness of individual strands.

d) The color and texture of hair.

Answer: a) The way hair absorbs and retains moisture.

3. Question

Which hair type is characterized by tight, coily curls that require more moisture retention techniques?

a) 2A

b) 3B

c) 4C

d) 1C

Answer: c) 4C

Lesson 3: Common Hair Myths and Misconceptions

1. Question

Which of the following is a common misconception about natural hair?

a) Natural hair grows slower than straight hair.

b) Natural hair cannot be versatile.

c) Natural hair is more prone to breakage.

d) All of the above.

Answer: d) All of the above.

2. Question

What is one science-based fact about natural hair?

a) Hair should be washed daily to prevent dryness.

b) Cutting hair more frequently makes it grow faster.

c) Natural oils produced by the scalp help keep hair moisturized.

d) Hair should always be straightened for it to grow.

Answer: c) Natural oils produced by the scalp help keep hair moisturized.

General Quiz on Module 1

1. Question

What role did natural hair play in the Civil Rights Movement?

a) It was seen as a form of protest and self-expression.

b) It was discouraged and hidden to fit societal norms.

c) It was associated with rebellion against the government.

d) It had no significant role during that period.

Answer: a) It was seen as a form of protest and self-expression.

2. Question

Why is understanding your curl pattern important for hair care?

a) It determines the type of products you should use.

b) It defines how often you should wash your hair.

c) It tells you how long your hair will grow.

d) It shows whether or not you should use heat styling tools.

Answer: a) It determines the type of products you should use.

CLOSING NOTE

You don't have to fight your hair anymore.

You just have to understand it.

This is where your journey *really* begins.